CW00664444

A Plan For Extirpating The Venereal Disease

You are holding a reproduction of an original work that is in the public domain in the United States of America, and possibly other countries.You may freely copy and distribute this work as no entity (individual or corporate) has a copyright on the body of the work.This book may contain prior copyright references, and library stamps (as most of these works were scanned from library copies).These have been scanned and retained as part of the historical artifact.

This book may have occasional imperfections such as missing or blurred pages, poor pictures, errant marks, etc. that were either part of the original artifact, or were introduced by the scanning process. We believe this work is culturally important, and despite the imperfections, have elected to bring it back into print as part of our continuing commitment to the preservation of printed works worldwide. We appreciate your understanding of the imperfections in the preservation process, and hope you enjoy this valuable book.

thoughts, which I addrefs to you in this form.

I am fenfible, that our friend the Dean † has in fome meafure antici-pated my project; but his fcheme carries with it fo very ludicrous an air, and is, in fome degree, fo extreamly impracticable, that I do not think my plan fhould be laid afide for want of novelty.

The Dean propofes to falivate the inhabitants of all Europe, the priefts of every denomination not excepted. Now, without this were abfolutely put in practice in every part, at one

---

† Swift.

and

and the fame time, it would be of no manner of fignification — as the inhabitants of Naples (to begin at the fountain-head) being falivated in January, they might be infected afrefh in February by the Lombardians, tho' even their females were prevented having any intercourfe with that people — and fo on: and the difficulty of falivating all Europe (the clergy not excepted) at the fame period, muft appear evident to the moft common obferver.

Nor do I hold it right, either phyfically or politically, to extirpate the venereal diforder entirely from the face of Europe ; for I do not know, whether the medicinal gentlemen might

not

not think it expedient, at fome particular periods, to import a certain quan-
tity of the Virus for innoculation, or
fome other cogent ufe ; which confideration I fhall attend to in my plan.
Then, again, whilft we remain fo
perfectly found in our body corporate,
we fhall add greatly to the *foundnefs*
of our body politic, by not only being a more healthy and robuft people
in general (you wont then fee fuch a
puny wretch as me once in a twelve-
month) and thereby greatly increafing
our wealth, as the fame number of
hands will be able to gain more, without the affiftance of foreigners, by
manufactures, labour, and agricul-
ture ; — but alfo by the fuccefs of our
arms, as we may expect they will then
be

be infinitely more fortunate than ever
they were, under even the great duke
of Marlborough ; for as one Englifh-
man, by the help of roaft-beef and
plumb-pudding, can now eafily beat
feven foup-meagre Frenchmen ; fo
then, doubtlefs, one found Englifh-
man, will be able to beat a dozen
rotten Frenchmen.

Thefe confiderations, phyfical and
political, but more particularly political, I intend to confine my plan of
deracinating the venereal diforder to
the ifland of Great-Britain only. The
reafon why I do not extend it to my
weftern compatriots the Irifh, is, I
muft acknowledge, infufed with fome-
thing of a national jealoufy, in a
point,

point, which for fo good a chriftian as
I am, has too much excited my jealoufy. But my Hibernian friends will
have this confolation, that let what
accident foever happen to them, by
the want of my plan taking place in
Ireland, they will always be upon a
par with us in this refpect. This may,
however, in fome meafure alleviate the
mortification I have always had, and
which every true Briton muft neceffarily have, to think that the inhabitants of a vice-royalty, or a feparated
province, fhould have one inch more
advantage in any particular, than the
natives of the mother-country. I dare
fay, my friend the dean, through a
certain national prejudice, which even
he cannot diveft himfelf of in all
points,

points, differs with me greatly in this refpect.

My fcheme, dear St. J—n, is in a few words this, that there be doctors and furgeons, whofe eminence and fkill are well attefted, appointed all over England and Wales, and alfo in Scotland, to examine and infpect parochially every refident, within the limits of each parifh.

That thefe phyfical gentlemen qualify themfelves alfo, by a prior and reciprocal examination, before a certain number of the moft learned of the quorum. That a proclamation be publifhed, ftrictly prohibiting *all procreation* whatever, during the fpace of

at

at leaſt ſix weeks; and as the holy
time of Lent is appointed for faſting,
this would be the propereſt period to
fix upon for the ſaid abſtinence, as a
reſtraint from fleſh would be a great
means of enabling the more laſcivious
and abandoned to quit their lewd and
wicked courſes, at leaſt for that time.

The preparatory celibacy having
taken place, as well as the ſubſequent
examination and inſpection, a proper
and faithful report ſhould be made of
the ſame, and ſuch public or private
places be appointed in every two
pariſhes, for thoſe patients, who were
found in any degree contaminated
with the diſorder, to undergo a proper
courſe of phyſic.

C   Of

Of every two parifhes, only one fhould be put into this courfe at a time, upon the fuppofition, that there would not be a fufficient number of wholefome people remaining in one parifh, and who condefcend to affift the infected during their purification. By this means the contiguous parifh might affift their neighbours during this period, and they, in turn, fhould be affifted by thefe. — At this time none fhould be admitted abroad, or allowed to procreate, till they had received a certificate, figned by the doctor or furgeon, who attended them, of their perfect fanity ; and even then be defended from any carnal conver-

fation,

iation, but with fuch as had received a like certificate.

This fcheme being general, it of courfe includes both males and females, laity as well as clergy, of all ranks and denominations. Notwithftanding this plan might be thus far exe-cuted, with the greateft care and pre-cifion, there might, neverthelefs, many objects efcape, either through their own ignorance, or that of their phyfician, or through the artifices of the one or the other : a law fhould therefore be enforced, that after a certain time limited, any man, however exalted, who communicated this diforder to a female, fhould be fined 10*l.* (as in the cafe of a baftard being laid to

C 2 him(

him) for the benefit of parish good-eating — this would make the parochial officers very attentive to their duty. The woman, from a dowager dutchefs, down to a baronet, or -alderman's lady, fhould pay the fame fum, under that quality 5*l.* That for the fecond offence they fhould ftand on the pillory; and if they fhould go fo far as a third offence, if a man, he fhould have the offending part cut off, as it is reafonable to fuppofe it, by this time, nearly in a ftate of amputation; if a woman, fhe fhould be divefted of all appearances of her fex, except for one particular function.

If

If thefe penalties and punifhments would not prevent the propagation of the diforder, from fome latent embers had efcaped extinguifhing ; other more exemplary punifhments might be inflicted—it might be made felony with as much juftice as the theft of a fhilling.

Having made thefe neceffary provifions for the deftruction of this diforder at home ; it would be neceffary to take fome precautions to prevent the importation of it from abroad. To this end, proper officers fhould be appointed, for the infpection of all perfons coming into this kingdom, who fhould not be admitted to land, with-

out

out having certificates of their health, or at leaft of their being exempt from this diforder.

I am not fo vain a projector, as to imagine, there can be no objections made to this my plan; but as the good of the community is always to be preferred to the intereft of individuals; and as alfo fome fcruples, which may at firft be made, may, with fome attention, be renewed, or at leaft weakened, I think this fcheme fhould not be entirely laid afide, for thefe confiderations. To evince what I fay, I fhall, myfelf, urge the moft plaufible and weighty objections that can be made to it, and fhall at the fame time endeavour to point out the means, if

not

not entirely to remove them, at leaſt to ſoften and render them more ſupportable.

The firſt important and formidable objection that offers, is the diminution of inhabitants that will be occaſioned, and the loſs that poſterity will ſuſtain, by a ſix weeks celibacy throughout Great-Britain. To this it may be anſwered, that the more than redoubled vigour, with which each individual will return to the charge, will at leaſt counterbalance this loſs ; as it is not the repetition or frequency of coition that produces children, but the lucky hit of a well muſtered roll, with mutual warm deſires worked up to their proper pitch, reciprocally and critically

tically gratified. If to this we add
the foundnefs of the offspring, and
their being exempted, not only from
all venereal taints, but alfo the leprofy,
the evil, and many other diforders,
which are its natural heirs; and that
thereby many thoufand lives will be
faved of the firft nine months pro-
duce.

I queftion whether the number of
the inhabitants will be reduced even
for the firft year; and that pofterity
muft be thereby greatly increafed, is,
I think, beyond a doubt; when it is
confidered how many millions of lives
muft only, in the courfe of a century,
be produced and faved, where they
otherwife would not, if this deftruc-

tive

tive diftemper were not exterminated from this ifland.

The next objection, which though it may not carry with it fo many marks of univerfal oppofition, may, neverthelefs, be more formidably fupported than the preceding; and from this fimple and right obfervation, " that what is every body's bufinefs is no body's; but what affects the feeming intereft of any particular body of men, will certainly meet with adverfaries, directly or indirectly, from that quarter." I prefume you already anticipate my meaning, and I have fcarce occafion to fubjoin, that thefe opponents are compofed of the phyfical, or rather the chirurgical part of

the

the world. I have already premifed, that the intereft of individuals íhould, upon all occafions, fubmit to the benefit of the community : to this I may add, that thefe gentlemen will, upon this occafion, enter into immediate and great practice, and many of them may accumulate large and inftantaneous fortunes, by this very fcheme's taking place. Thofe whofe merit may be overlooked, with regard to prefent practice, and whofe dependence may, in fome meafure, be upon the continuation of the progrefs of the venereal virus, will certainly be able to make friends to obtain appointed infpectors at the fea-ports, as we cannot fuppofe common excifemen fo able to fwear to the genuine-

nefs

nefs of the French diforder, as French brandy. Befides, if after this there fhould be any phyfical or chirurgical men unprovided for, I have left a door open for the neceffary importation of this commodity, duty free, at any convenient period.

I muft acknowledge that the ladies (I mean the ladies of pleafure) would have a more reafonable plea to oppofe this plan, if this very plan was not fo replete with advantageous confequences to them. — To explain this feeming paradox; it would be very hard upon thefe, to be obliged to fhut up their *fhops* for fix weeks, when, perhaps, they may have but a fmall ftock in *hand*, if many benefits would not

flow

flow to them from it in the *end.* I say, it would be very cruel for thefe poor females, to be obliged to faft and pray all Lent (which is generally their greateft harveft, by reafon of there being fewer public diverfions) and be debarred, perhaps, fifh as well as flefh (fprats their common food not excepted) if they did not thereby purge their fouls as well as bodies — avoid all future diforders fo incidental to their trade, and go on fwimmingly ever-after, without the interruption of one fingle falivation. — Befides, if, during thefe fix weeks, they do not gain the ufual profits of their calling, they are at no expence to fubfift (as thefe women, at leaft, being fo public, fhould be cured at the public charge) and

may,

may, therefore, fancy they were asleep
all that time, or passed a night with a
charitable bilk.

If there should be any *real* ladies
so far *priest-ridden*, as to believe it were
too heinous a sin to discontinue the
propagation of their species for six
weeks; or, being of too delicate a
texture to undergo the visitation of a
man upon so obscene an occasion,
some provisios might be made in their
favour; for instance, they might, in
the first case, being upon a fair examination pronounced *found*, be allowed to procreate for the benefit of man-
kind, after ten days abstinence; and
this they could not think any very
great vacation, since the Jewish ladies,

upon

upon another occafion, are compelled once a month to a fortnight's celibacy; — but thefe we are to fuppofe Chriftian ladies; and, therefore, this Jewifh regulation may have but little weight with them. In the fecond cafe, thefe tender females might have every part of their bodies hidden, but the moft natural; without we could fuppofe them very malignantly infected, which, though not entirely impoffible, would be extreamly incompatible with their extraordinary delicacy. However this, or fome fuch *indulgence*, might prevent their modefty being offended at the obfcenity of a male infpection, particularly if they had ever been lain by a man-midwife.

The

The clergy, though a very difinterefted fet of men, might, from fome *religious* motive, oppofe it ; Firft, As during the fix weeks celibacy no marriages would be folemnized ; and, Secondly, As it might alfo, in fome meafure, prevent them for the future, by reafon of the dangers which now flow from a general commerce with the fex being in a great meafure prevented. If the firft objection had any other foundation than the lofs that would accrue to the church, by the ceremonial fees not taking place during that period ; it might be anfwered upon the fame principle, as the objection made with regard to the diminution of inhabitants, and the lofs

thereby

thereby occasioned to posterity. And I think the latter objection,' however religiously cloathed, proves so good an argument for my plan, that I can never give the health and satisfaction of my countrymen up, on the supposition of its preventing some foolish matches, which would be productive of nothing but beggary; and, in the end, incumbrances to the parishes in which they were solemnized. As to such prudential and reasonable marriages, which are the proper cement of society, they can never be diminished, or detrimented, by this, or any other plan that promotes the benefit of the common-weal. This is giving the argument its greatest latitude — greater than, upon a proper scrutiny,

can

can be admitted, and yet we fee of
how little force it is; or rather how
much it proves the utility of the
fcheme. But can it ferioufly be be-
lieved, that men are fo foolifh, as to
be frightened into marriage, through
the fear of being infected with this
diforder; or that they are a whit more
fecure in this ftate, than if they re-
mained conftant to any one woman,
without the connubial ceremony having been performed.

Perhaps it may be afked, from
whence a fufficient fund is to arife
to pay the expence of the execution
of this project, and particularly to
make a proper recompence to the faculty, for their immediate attendance,

E   and

and their future loffes ? I have already had occafion to hint, that the expence which the ladies of pleafure fhould occafion this way, fhould neceffarily and equitably fall upon the public, to whom they were indebted for their misfortunes. This naturally leads us to confider of a tax, to raife a proper fum for the general fcheme. I fhould imagine it could not coft two millions fterling, to falivate all the inhabitants of Great-Britain as were in a defperate way, and make an ample provifion for the gentlemen of the faculty ; efpecially, as it is to be hoped it would not be neceffary to reduce above one third of the inhabitants to that extremity ; and as the other courfes of phy-
fic

ne and regimens neceffary would not amount to any very confiderable fum.

Suppofing this calculation to be founded in fact, this neceffary fum might, methinks, be eafily and very equitably produced, by a tax upon — Nofes. Surely no man would think it a burthenfome impoft, to pay one guinea for the fecurity of the nofe on his face ; and I hope there are at leaft a fourth part of the inhabitants of this ifland, that have this ornamental fea-ture remaining. There could be no cheating the revenue in this refpect, and the manner of collecting the tax would be very plain.

E 2   Having

Having made the neceffary provifion for carrying this plan into execution, it may be needlefs to point out
the means of paying the officers or
chirurgical infpectors appointed at the
fea-ports, as the paffes which they
would grant to fuch as came from
abroad in health, might be raifed for
their benefit.

I know but one body of people remaining, who can with any face oppofe my project: — thcfe are the
coach-makers †. I have heard it com-
puted,

---

† 1 was going to add the peruke-makers —
but upon reflexion, I fuppofe, the gentlemen of
the

puted, that there are at leaſt one hun-
dred chariots rolling about London,
upon gallipots and boluſſes ; and it
would be in vain to hide the truth,
the venereal diſorder has no ſmall ſhare
in this circulation ; ſo that I cannot
ſuppreſs my apprehenſions, that ſome
of theſe charioteers may become *foot-*
men. — I do not mean according to
the common acceptation, of the
which capacity they now officiate lite-
rally, upon every door-opening occa-
ſion. I foreſaw the loſſes the coach-
makers would ſuſtain, and I acknowledge them ; and at the ſame time

---

the faculty will continue wearing — their volumi-
nous perukes, they are ſo ornamental.

that

that I am not fchemift fufficient at this juncture, to devife any means for, making them a proper recompence — without it be, that they and their wives, their daughters, their maids, and, in fhort, all their families, as far as their firft coufins (and no farther) be *falivated*, if fo they fhould require, *gratis*, and without any of them paying the nofe-tax, though each and every one of them be embellifhed with that prominent and graceful feature.

Having fhewn this plan of mine to an intimate acquaintance, when I had got thus far, he inffifted upon it, that *nofes* fhould pay in proportion to their length; and he does not think my

scheme

fcheme will be entirely effectual without monkies are included; but this I
fhall leave to the confideration of thofe
who may chufe to improve upon my
plan.

I would not have you, dear St.
J—n, by what I have faid, fuppofe I
intend to include in my fcheme, the
extirpation of the intellectual gonor-
rhœa; fo far from this, I would not
pretend to perform one fingle radical
cure in this diforder, which I look
upon as altogether beyond the phyfician's fkill. The utmoft I can do,
will be to point out the fymptoms of
this difeafe, that the uninfected may
fhun the contagious; and firft let me
caution every one, who would efcape

being

being infected, to carefully avoid a certain set of ladies, whose company is nine times more dangerous than that of all the rest of the sex put together.

Upon first affociating with thefe females, one is very apt to be hideoufly troubled with that naftly difor-der, called the *cacoethes fcribendi* — this generally brings on an *oozing of the brain* ‡, which is moft commonly

attended

---

‡ The moft celebrated authors that have wrote upon this fubject, differ greatly in this point : He-roditius Suetonicus is of this opinion ; but Sa-peritius Caput pofitively avers, that this difcharge is from a watery head ; and fupports this opinion, by his own *anatomical practice,* in the courfe of

which

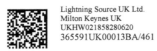

Lightning Source UK Ltd.
Milton Keynes UK
UKHW021858280620
365591UK00013BA/461